IN TOUCH
WITH
REIKI II

In Touch with Reiki II

A Manual
for Teachers and Students

Usui Reiki II

~

Susan Rea Caldwell
Master/Teacher

Usui Reiki II
Copyright 2007
by Susan Rea Caldwell
4creatingpaths@gmail.com

ISBN: 978-1-542-8336-9-1

~

Susan Rea Caldwell holds a Masters Degree in English. She has published many short stories and two novels, Joseph's Journey and Betty Rea and Tales from smack in the middle of New Hampshire Drive and Beyond. She has been awarded several artist grants from the Kentucky Foundation for Women. She is a labyrinth builder and facilitator certified through Veriditas. She leads creative workshops including Julia Cameron's The Artist's Way. She is Master/Teacher in Usui Reiki and an Akashic Records Consultant through ARCI.

Anything and everything stated in this workbook is from the experience of Susan Caldwell. It is meant to give you, the reader, the student of Reiki, guidelines. Accept and reject at your own discretion.
Follow your own truth, your own path.
Be true to your Source and yourself above all else.

~ Dedication ~

This book is dedicated to all of my Reiki students without whom a Master/Teacher would not be necessary. I honor your commitment to studying Reiki and expanding your knowledge and use of Reiki energy.

The information in this book references healing which is a different discipline than medicine. I in no way offer medical advice or wish to discredit the medical community in any way. In case of serious illness consult your physician.

I trust our endeavors bring a more peaceful existence to ourselves, our friends, family, and colleagues. I believe our efforts will bring peace and joy to our planet and beyond.

I applaud you for you are a beautiful soul and the Light of the Creator shines through YOU.

Note to the Reader:

I will interchange the titles Source, Universe, God, Spirit, and Creator throughout this document. As Reiki has no religious connections, the energy used is Life Force Energy. I mean to connect with no particular religion here, however, my background is Christian, and I do not deny my basis and strength in this particular dogma. I mean no offense in any words or lack of wording. I believe Source to be above religion and inclusive of ALL – all life. I believe we all are one and come from one Source.

~ Table of Contents ~

~ 1 ~
Blessing the monetary exchange

As I am one with God, I am one with my God,
for God is both the Giver and the Gift.
I cannot separate the Giver from the Gift.
Shin, *The Game of Life and How to Play It,* 94.

In our society we place value on something that is important to us and our life choices. The value of the exchange is measured typically by money. It is an honor for me to accept money in exchange for this Reiki II attunement. The sacredness of the passing of the attunements sets the energy for the ceremony. It allows the exchange of goods to take place. When the money is blessed for mind, body, and spirit it brings all aspects together for the betterment, the goodness and the highest exchange for all concerned.

The student offering money verifies their choice to learn Reiki, to awaken to becoming a more loving person, to be more in control of his or herself, and to grow spiritually on their unique journey.

In turn, the Reiki Master/Teacher exchanges their knowledge and perspective, their understanding, and gifts through Reiki. Because of the attunement lineage, this exchange filters through each and every Reiki student/teacher.

I will barter a partial payment with a Reiki attunement but not the entire price. I believe the ingrained value of money has an aspect that cannot be ignored. And I do not wish for money to hinder or stop a person's desire to learn. I will say that 95% of the Reiki attunements that I have gifted, Reiki is not used or practiced by that recipient!

When the person hands me the payment, I hold it in my hands in a prayer position and ask that the money return to them tenfold. I provide a vase or jar to place the money in for the rest of the class.

I then welcome each student to the highest of their unique and individual good. To learn. To co-create. To be the best their Creator meant them to be. By saying yes with love to Reiki I, the student honors himself or herself, the teacher, and the planet.

THANK YOU, the reader, for inviting me to join you and to guide you on this occasion and in this sacred connection of our journeys.

~ **2** ~

Introduction

Reiki II is an intensification of Reiki I from the standpoint that this attunement increases the intensity of the vibrations moving through your body, allowing for a stronger, more focused energy and a more profound spiritual connection. It has been likened to mathematically squaring Reiki I.

This level brings with it the introduction of three of Usui Reiki's five sacred symbols. The symbols may be familiar to you, or they may not be, but each carries connections to intense healing energies or capabilities. They have been passed down for centuries through Reiki attunements. They are used in the attunement process to open the energy flow and strengthen healing capabilities when called upon in a healing session.

One particular symbol, the Hon-Sha-Ze-Sho-Nen, is used to send distance Reiki which is like a prayer with a focused intention. Thus, the intention of the thought must be pure. In other words, the concept of removing oneself from another's situation and incorporating the oneness of All in healing becomes the primary intention. The All-Is-One experience will become more and more the platform from which you will speak and promote yourself and your healing. Understanding the interconnectedness of all life forms will become a part of your experience. Incorporating this concept causes the collapse of linear time, thus creating the plausibility of healing in the past as well as the present and into the future. So, pure projections become vital in changing the events and the situations in the lives of yourself and those with whom you work. The responsibility of this is huge and it is karmic. With these symbols and this capability, we deal with soul issues, and this is a responsibility not to be taken lightly.

This is my belief. Herein lies a language I have found to express my truth after having many conversations and reading shelves of books and participating in myriads of Reiki sessions and prayer groups. If this is not your truth, then you will find opportunities to reconcile and incorporate your individual beliefs into your Reiki system.

Remember that Reiki energy cannot harm. By using Reiki to fit into the highest and best good for all concerned, we bring healing possibilities to every situation, every person, and everything because of the ripple affect one has upon another, and another, and another.

For example, if someone is going to surgery, ask for "the person and all concerned" to receive a blessing. This way, in addition to blessing the patient, we are assured that the surgeon, the nursing staff, the cleanup crew, and the family are also blessed. And if they all accept the blessing (which by the law of free will, they can choose to refuse) then they carry on that blessing to those whose lives they touch. The blessing grows much like a spider's web. The prayer at the center works its way outward in many directions, expanding and expanding.

I love the exercise of blessing my food and everyone who has come in contact with it since its inception. I often bless all the cars that pass me on the road. I like to come up with something expansive like, "Thank you God, for blessing everyone wearing denim today." Be generous with your prayers and thoughts. Be creative. God can handle it and, I believe, your rewards will return multiplied in ways you cannot imagine.

The Reiki lineage itself is a blessing. It is a miraculous bond with other Reiki healers and beings of similar interests and intentions. They will become your network. Spirit Guides are also anxious to escort you on your way. They are anxious for healing to take place. An interesting meditation is to send Reiki to a past Master. A woman I know receives guidance from Mrs. Takata and I have been visited and assisted by the spirit of Dr. Usui in individual healings and during the attunement processes.

Ask your Guides to reveal themselves, to guide you. Expect to become more familiar with them. Their presence will become more evident as your intuitive channels clear and open. Thank your healing Guides often for their guidance, devotion, and unconditional love. Marianne Williamson says we do not ask for enough. And remember the adage, watch what you pray for, you just might get it! So, expect to receive what you desire. Visualize it. Feel it.

In book one of Conversations with God, God says, "Every prayer – every thought, every statement, every feeling – is creative. To the degree that it is fervently held at truth, to that degree will it be made manifest in your experience." (p 12). Use gratitude as a method of prayer instead of want. Any supplication including "want" creates just that – a situation of want. Pray in thanksgiving not as a request.

Look for and expect more synchronicity in your life to guide and direct you. Miracles, you may choose to call them. You will be in closer touch with the spiritual universe and should expect this openness to aid you along your life's journey. Divine synchronicity can be as simple as a phone call from a person you just thought about; something more complex like a workshop being canceled and you are available to attend another one of greater importance. It could be something like the book you would like to read is back ordered and a friend shows up with it the next day. Coincidence, we tend to call it. Or is it an ever-adjusting path of less resistance and opportunity unfolding as a result of those hard working synchronicity Angels?

Clearing after a Reiki II initiation should bring much the same physical experiences as the Reiki I, with the addition of emotional issues that will surface. Situations in your everyday life will mirror those which are surfacing. See these events as signals, as current reminders that give you parallels to assist you in your work to become unblocked and untangled and find enlightenment on your spiritual journey. See them as the Universe saying pay attention!

As a Reiki II your energy will become cleaner, purer. This is not a statement to say that others have dirty energy or unpure energy, but that your energetic field is cleansing through the process of accessing this higher vibration and others will want to share it. And ... because Reiki insists that you attend to the work of the Inner you, you will become a beacon, a seeker searching for self-truth. As a result, people, whether they are aware of it or not, may tend to cling to you more and try to take energy from you. Remember the energy-sucking person in James Redfield's Celestine Prophecy? Protect yourself from these people who take without balance, without permission. Do not allow yourself to be depleted by their stories, dramas or time demands. You have worked hard to get where you are, treasure your growth. Respect your position. Protect yourself. Share with anyone with whom you feel so inclined, offer your vision and a map to anyone requesting directions, but be wary of those who want a free ride. "Allow each soul to walk its path," (CWG, p 47).

With Reiki II you are more adept, more prepared to send Reiki out, to give Reiki. One Reiki Master recommends that just her Reiki II's do sessions on others, not her level I's. She says that because level II's are more opened to the vibration of the energy, more opened to intuitive understanding, and have been introduced to the symbols and their specific healing traits, they are better equipped to put their hands on others. I, however, believe any Reiki channeled through any level is better than none. Either belief, I encourage you to consider involving more people, inviting others to share the wonder of Reiki. I feel like a missionary of sorts, like I am a merchant with good "vibes" to share. I believe that the more positive energy that is placed out there, the more the positives will grow. So, the more you use your Reiki, the better our world will be.

For this reason, I suggest then that you participate in Reiki shares on a regular basis for self-healing and creating a network of like minds. Creating a forum gives participants a place to explore, to exchange ideas. It becomes a safe haven, a school room for learning and experiencing the many doors Reiki can unlock. And as you use your Reiki the more polished your vessel becomes. A Reiki share can be two coming together to lay hands on each other or many who come to give and receive healing energy.

You may be called to become so involved with Reiki that you wish to set up a practice. For this reason, I have included some practical information on facilitating a balance. Check out other practitioner's healing spaces to find what you like and do not like. Create your own special space for you and your healing mission. You will be guided by the Divine and be supported.

Like the puppy outside my window chasing a leaf, enjoy your Reiki. Use it creatively. If you are a student, bless your books and the pencil you take notes with. If you are scheduled to make a speech, bless the podium, the room, and the audience. Reiki your doctor's office and the nurse's hands. Do not forget your animals and plants. Reiki your medicine, your vitamins, your shoes when you go out into the rain! Your car. The phone when a telemarketer calls. Jesus asked us to bless our enemy. Expand your blessings to include healing for those you disagree with, those who make you angriest, and those you fear. For healing's sake.

Our world can use healing in every direction, on all levels. Turn on your Reiki and allow healing energy to flow in, around and through you.

I have a friend who, in high school, wanted to save the world – really. This was in late 60s. She graduated from our all white, southern high school, got pregnant with her African American boyfriend and was immediately disowned by her family. She moved two miles away, just across the river and by herself earned a degree in nursing while raising her boy. The young man is a fine person. He is kind and caring. Everyone who meets him is forced to look at any bias they carry about race and family and gender. I saw even the most racist person forced to admit they like this mother and son. And you know what? My friend did save the world. Her area of the world. Because she did the best she knew how. She fiercely loved her son and raised him, and she had so much love to share she became a nurse. She took the situation and made it livable. By living her truth with compassion and determination she opened the hearts of many.

You too can change the world. Your world. For you are a safe, sacred, and successful Reiki healer. And by healing yourself you do heal the world.

Any student of Reiki considering working on other people should check their local requirements about touching another person's body. I am a licensed minister through the Universal Brotherhood. Being a minister allows me permission in the state of Kentucky to touch another person's body, perform marriages and funerals and to enter ICU.

I am insured to protect myself and the establishment where I have a Reiki studio.

Use your Reiki.

~ 3 ~
# Clearing

Clearing after a Reiki II initiation should bring much the same physical experiences as that of level I. Flu symptoms, stomach "stuff." Sweating, an aversion to noise and clutter and extraneous goings on. Nothing water and Reiki cannot adjust. However, with Reiki II the addition of emotional issues will surface, because you are called to become more responsible for your emotional and mental attitudes. To justify them. To clear them of what is not your truth. To respond to and affect every thought, action, word, and deed that comes to your being.

Diane Stein says to expect emotional issues to surface for the next six months and urges us to trust that the issues will not appear until we are ready for them.

If happy or joyous emotions reveal themselves, revel in their occurrence and bask in their pleasure. If not-so-happy ones surface, know that the Universe is presenting these tough ones to you. The issues may be ones you are already aware of or thought you had addressed. They may be ones long buried because they were too painful to deal with at the time. They may be brand new! See any exposed emotions as a door opening, as a starting point on a road to wellness, as a place to begin healing. Reiki energy allows for few secrets and will allow you to release your issues layer by layer as you are ready to deal with each.

Are you afraid what you will dredge up will be too painful?

Trust in the knowledge that you will not be given more than you can handle and understand that you now have access to a more intense self-healing energy. Plus, you are more in communication with your Angels and Spirit Guides, and you have access to the three symbols to apply in appropriate situations. The Hon-Sha-Ze-Sho-Nen is one of the symbols you will learn to use with this attunement. It is powerful and it will help to heal and harmonize past, present, and future.

Reiki will provide the coping abilities to deal with the issues presented. Do not brush the emotions aside as being pointless. Do not fear what you are presented. Do not anger at events of the past. They can no longer hurt you and have not surfaced to inflict pain, but to initiate healing. Trust that whatever situations arise, they are there for you to look at without fear of further pain, existing to soothe and mend and repair and heal. "The past is over; it can touch me not" is an excellent lesson from *A Course in Miracles* which makes a perfect mantra (442).

Outside situations in your everyday life will mirror those which are surfacing from the inside. See these situations around you as self-reflecting opportunities for healing. After all, we can only "fix" ourselves and to do so, don't we need to see the problems?

When these mirrors appear re-act with your new knowledge, your new "take" on things. Investigate the theater of life that surrounds you and take what you want from your movie and proceed. Heal your life. Co-create your universe.

The following is an e-mail I received after a first level Reiki attunement:

"I've been meaning to write to you for a while, I just can't seem to find time to sit down and do it. I just wanted you to know that I've been doing fine. I've remembered things that you said to me & Linda about dealing with other people & customers at work, [I suggested she see everything as an opportunity to learn and grow

in herself, and to see others as fellow, loving, struggling souls.] and I wanted you to know that it's really made a difference. I don't know how to explain this, but I feel different since my attunement. It's like I'm calmer, empowered, freer or something. Things that used to would have really gotten on my nerves, just sort of slide off me now. I don't feel like the world is my responsibility. I've been doing little things that probably would seem silly to other people, but to me they are huge in that they give me a since of self power. For instance, if I see a recipe that sounds good, I just get the stuff and make it for dinner instead of asking my husband if he would like to try it. If he doesn't like it, I figure he'll heat up a bowl of soup or something. If I know that I need to run a few errands after work or grab a bite to eat before going home, I leave the boys at daycare a little longer and go do what I need to do instead of rushing straight to pick them up and trying to juggle everything and keep them happy at the same time. I feel calmer and not so stressed when I do these things. I feel like I am taking care of me first, and that is helping me to take care of my family better. I'm also getting better at telling people no. I love it. I feel powerful.

I honestly feel like I'm entering a new chapter in my life. It's hard to explain. It's like things have been reprioritized. I feel more centered toward family and not so much toward work. I'm figuring out what makes me happy and not what would make other people happy. I just wanted to let you know that you helped to awaken some hidden part of my brain or something. It's like I've changed course or something. Now, don't get me wrong, I do not have everything figured out yet, but I feel like I have new tools to help me get there."

Say your Reiki principals often. Bless the surfacing events for bringing you the situation to mend and grow. Begin the process by forgiving the situation itself, yourself as a participant and anyone else involved. Forgiveness is often not something that happens overnight, but the first step is to say, "I forgive." Even if the words sound hollow at first, repeat them and feel them resonate and start to dislodge ingrained thoughts.

19

Do not neglect to forgive yourself. Explore any residual guilt and pain you may be harboring as roots to your current beliefs. Include attitudes towards yourself, your spirituality, your relationships, and so on. In looking inward, do your actions and attitudes differ from your core truths, the truths you hold in your heart as to your authentic self? Witnessing our positives is easy. Witnessing our negatives, not so much. Seeing what we've created for ourselves and others is often not a warm fuzzy! Looking at ourselves with all of our limitations and baggage is not an easy task. Love your soul, forgive your physical, emotional, and mental self. Introduce and make peace with the four bodies (physical, mental, emotional, and spiritual) that make up who you are. Live as one entity in purpose and mission. You cannot do this if the four are in conflict or if one body is saying the other is wrong. Call a truce. Forgive yourself and **LOVE YOURSELF**. To thy own self be true.

One way to free yourself from painful memories is to hand them over to your Higher Power. Some do this by writing through the experience and the feelings associated with the person and/or situation and then burn the paper in a symbolic place like in the garden or under a favorite tree. Or sail them down a river or stream. Remember that the more senses you include in the process the stronger the influence of what you are doing is on the mental body. If you speak the release, you hear it. If you write it down, you can feel it and touch what you are processing. The more sensory attributes you use the deeper your whole self is involved.

Send the situation off with as little negativity as possible. Bless the release even if you are not 100% convinced of any or all of the blessings the event has brought to your experience. Visualize your personal trauma turning into something positive. Ashes or note paper can become fertilizer for your favorite rose bush. Ask for loving healing light to bless everyone, everything involved. Do not limit the healing to yourself. Include all involved.

Another visualization: Pack a memory suitcase with the reminiscences of what you are trying to release with a thousand rose pedals. Send them to a perfume factory where they are turned in to a luscious, passionate scent. Be creative.

When I first began this forgiveness process, I visualized Jesus with a basket and as my thoughts and fears surfaced I'd fill up His basket. (This brings a Christian, Biblical resonance to using Reiki, but it is in my background, and you are free to use or dismiss this as your heart directs whether or not you profess Christianity as part of your belief system.) I believe any loving deity would do the same for you. The struggle became putting myself in the basket! Or Self-forgiveness.

Think about this: What if there is no good and bad? No right and wrong? What if there are only situations that present opportunities for us to aspire to love without conditions, without judgments? What if situations are presented for us to aspire to seeing others as the loving being that is their true soul?

Use your Reiki to face any discomfort that arises. See it from the aspect of a visitor, a third party. You do not have to be in the situation again, just focus on the problem. Be the observer. From which chakra does the discomfort originate? Do you need more solid footing, more creativity, more love, deeper spiritual insight? Work on that particular chakra. Wear clothing of the corresponding color. Reiki the journal you write in, the pencil, the keyboard, the computer desk. Reiki your pillow if your dreams get bad. Light white candles of purity and clearing. Sing the symbols. Dance for release. Walk in nature. There are hundreds of books that deal with release. They are written by people with much more knowledge than I have. Explore the possibilities. It may take more than one or two tries, one or two methods. Release is a process of letting go and the letting go most often happens in layers. One at a time. And the good news is that it is an ongoing process. We believe every physical distress is a result of clearing in some way. This can range from the flu to a migraine to a tooth ache or broken bone.

As you clean out your past debris, your collective background becomes a safe place and you will be free to frolic through your rediscovered, exposed areas carefree as a child, liberated from negative emotional baggage. This will allow your intuition to grow stronger and your relationship with your spiritual self to grow. Your truth will emerge easier. You will be able to look without the burden of fear, able to view every situation and every soul with love, with unconditional love. This is a difficult task without sound foundational moorings. You now have them. Reiki will support you.

Notice also any particular physical pain that develops with your second-degree clearing. Study how belief can influence biological symptoms. Louise Hay's *Heal Your Body* is an excellent reference text. So are Lise Bourbeau's texts. Never hesitate to see a doctor if you have an inkling that something is wrong, or you have put off that checkup way too long.

I do not in anyway, here or ever, disregard or discredit doctors or the traditional Western medical field. My daughter is an MD practicing family medicine. My brother and brother-in law, my aunt, and my cousin are nurses. I believe there are many paths to healing and that these myriads of choices offer diverse methods of coverage of all healing possibilities and combinations.

Bless this time as an opportunity to get your body back to emotional and physical wholeness. Bring your physical and emotional fears from darkness to light. Fill any voids with light and love. Empty dark areas and refill them with light.

You are the collective of all the events that have occurred in your life. It is your responsibility to use the events for your own good and the good of the others involved.

I also suggest keeping a journal. Write down your experiences. If you write every day, your experiences will begin to take some shape and the patterns will become congruent in a way you can recognize and work with them more effectively. In *The Artist's Way*, Julia Cameron suggests three pages every morning, 20-30 minutes, written in a stream of consciousness. The opportunities you are working through will then reveal themselves as just opportunities, not as the fickle finger of fate. This deepens your understanding of a co-creative universe. You will begin to see yourself less as a victim or floundering member of the human race. Figure how to co-create your universe.

Create happiness and joy and love.
Find it in every situation you encounter.
Learn it.
Live it.

~ 4 ~
Distance Reiki

The **Hon-Sha-Ze-Sho-Nen** to which you are being vibrationally attuned will enable you to send Reiki across distances. This ability is a blessing because the intention and healing can travel without need of a physical body. This is why I got my second level attunement. I wanted to be able to send Reiki to my loved ones. It is a prayer of sorts with a distinct energy attached to it.

To send the Reiki, have a pillow or teddy bear or some object to place your hands on. You may manipulate the object you hold in your hand as though the person's physical body is present. For example, move your hands down the teddy bear's chakras or just leave your hands steady and unmoving on a particular injury. Putting your hands on yourself is okay, but in my own experience, having a distinct object on which to focus the energy helps my concentration. A picture is helpful. Any visualization of the person or situation is also helpful. Remember those written pages I spoke of useful in clearing? They fit well into the palm of your hand for healing. Your absolute, undivided attention is not necessary, but it is helpful in developing your intuitive abilities and in learning to read the energy and the patterns. Reiki will find and work its way to the concern no matter how you develop your distance healing patterns.

I like to send distance Reiki at night before I go to sleep so I give the energy a specific amount of time to run, 30-60 minutes. I also like to send it while driving along long stretches of interstate where I am free to let my thoughts flow around the object of the healing.

To send distance Reiki I suggest:

1) State your intention. *My intention is to heal.*

2) Have permission from the recipient. This can be a verbal or spiritual agreement. Never force Reiki upon a person. Sending it without permission is not good spiritual manners. If you have not discussed Reiki with the person, ask their Spirit Guides. *Ask that the recipient receive the Reiki of their own free will and that the energy be used for the person's highest and best good.*

3) Give the energy a place to go in case the person refuses it. Send Reiki to the nearest river to help heal the industrial pollution we have inflicted. Leave the Reiki in the room or for the next person who enters and is willing to accept. Send it to the spouse abuse center, to the ICU waiting room, the neo-natal unit of your local hospital. Be creative.

4) Draw the Hon-Sha-Ze-Sho-Nen in your mind or visualize it. Say it three times. This symbol activates the vibrational mechanism for travel. You will feel the heat in your hands, the vibration. Use other symbols as you feel necessary.

5) Guide the energy. Ask that the energy heal on all levels. *Ask that the energy be used for the highest and best good of all concerned.* Do not try to direct the energy, just guide it. You are a conduit, a channel, not a director. Energies far more intelligent than we are doing the directing. (Thankfully!)

You can send Reiki with specific time conditions. You can do the Reiki healing at night for it to take effect the next day or at a past situation! Reiki time is not linear or sequential. Determine the time and place. (Diane Stein cautions against sending Reiki at the exact time of a surgery because it may affect the anesthesia. However, I do not believe Reiki can cause harm in any instance.) Ask that the person receive Reiki when applicable, when they go to sleep or during a doctor's appointment or during surgery. We sent so much Reiki to one woman's dentist appointment that the chair broke during the treatment. A friend who has panic attacks in hospitals was scheduled for surgery at 12:30. She says that she arrived at the hospital anxious but at 12:20 a great peace surrounded her, and she was calm and accepting and trusting.

Know that Reiki works. If you are sending the energy without the recipient being aware, please exercise caution. In my 2nd level exuberance, I substituted Reiki for my morning blessings to my children. One daughter called to say she'd had this weird diarrhea she couldn't explain, but wasn't sick, just "going." I humbled at the power of Reiki and backed off.

One woman who visits nursing homes to share her reflexology and Reiki with the residents questions her Reiki working consistently. "My hands get hot on some people and not on others." First remember that hot hands do not equal Reiki. Hot hands are not the demarcation. Hands may feel cold for inflammation or a headache. Some practitioner's hands do not ever get hot. Some are like heating pads. Draw your conclusions from the recipient's standpoint. The recipient is in charge. All we can do, as the channel, is offer.

We cannot force the Reiki or direct it. Accepting the healing energy is up to the person on the other side of your hands! Sometimes that is a tough lesson for us. We want to "fix it" for everyone, but each one of us has our lessons and experiences and we have no right to step between someone and their learning.

If a person does not want healing, we can't force it. Understand that we cannot make another's decisions for them. Each person is on their own journey, and it is unfair for us to take on their lessons. If a person does not accept Reiki and you are feeling frustrated because you think Reiki would be the best thing for them, do not force it.

To insert my personal religious beliefs here, I suggest you send prayer asking that s/he accept the healing light of God, the Source, the All-there-is, the Creator (what or whoever you believe is the force of life) that surrounds them. I believe we are all creations of God and are created with His/Her energy, thus our life-force is a "piece of," a segment of God and is ever present. So rather than ask that the love and/or light of God come to them and surround them, ask that they accept the healing light that is already there. God's constant love and light surrounds us awaiting an invitation. Also pray for yourself, that you are a right and perfect messenger, that words and wisdom come to you, that the right and perfect situation come to you to help guide the person in their healing process. Pray for the path and it will be lighted for you.

There are many web sites for Reiki practitioners and groups. Many offer distance healings for free or for a small charge. I urge you to look at these and take advantage of their services and perhaps offer your own.

Also, William Rand, a Reiki Master/teacher, in Michigan has placed a crystal at the North and South Pole for healing this planet. He will send you a picture of this crystal for you to send distance Reiki to it in an effort to promote world peace. Or get a little key chain globe. Send your Reiki for world peace. The planet we save just may be our own!

~ 5 ~
Why do Reiki healers get sick?

Physician, heal thyself.

One of the grandest benefits of the Reiki system is that the healing energy running through can and will affect the healer as well as the healee.

Is every illness a clearing? Opinions differ. I do believe we can clear any and all disease and distress from the physical body depending on the karmic attachment and the dedication to the process. I believe we are stronger than viruses and bacteria. I believe that with difficult, long standing cases, the healing takes longer. It takes work, lots of work, maybe even delving into past life issues, exploring all aspects of the many influences of disease. But I believe it can be done and I never discount the possibility of miracles.

As high vibrational beings, we must become more aware of consistent protection. Whenever necessary put yourself into what I call The Golden Glad Bag! Visualize yourself stepping into a white field of energy and tie it off at the top. See the protection from the bottoms of your feet upwards to a foot or so above your crown chakra. Remember to be aware of the effects of crowds, of people who are draining, and from whatever outside influences cause you concern.

Testing, checking the chakras, front and back, each morning

and night will help. Stating your intentions during the check should regulate them appropriately. This can be done by feeling them or reading them during meditation. The chakra energy should spiral or twist in your palm. If you cannot feel its spin snap your fingers in front of each one. A sharp snap will mean the chakra is open. A dull snap will mean closed. Testing this way, you can go back with your palm and feel the energy flow and learn how to pick up the sensation through your palm chakra. To open a closed chakra, rotate your hand while moving it away from the body.

When meditation time is available, sit in stillness and bring in the white light. Visualize it going down and through each chakra. Or meditate on the colors of the individual chakras noting any difficulty in bringing forth the colors as a way of identifying and correcting flow.

A short cut is to fluff the aura. Like combing your hair or wrapping yarn. Move your hands 2-3 feet out through your aura to keep the layers from collapsing against one another. Combing moves encroachments out and through, keeping other people's "stuff" from settling in, keeping what you are releasing from stopping anywhere on its way out, releasing blockages before they get to the physical body.

After working with a client whose release has been painful, emotional, or caused any great surge of release, remember to separate your heart chakra as you break from their energy field.

This can be done by drawing the Raku, the lightning bolt symbol in front of you from the third eye to the heart area. The Raku is a symbol used in passing attunements that separates the auric fields of the Reiki Master and the student. While you are not attuned to the third level of Reiki and cannot access the symbol to pass an attunement, the symbol has been used in your attunement and is in your energy field. Because of this, I believe it will work for you if your intention is to separate the auric fields of healer and healee.

I find this process necessary if the release is something that has been stored for a long time, like an old, painful emotional blockage. Work in people's auras and another's "stuff" leaves us vulnerable for that "stuff" to settle in our own. There are many ways to cleanse your energetic field. Wash your hands after every healing or run them atop a candle flame. Ground the energy by holding your palms parallel to the earth and see your energy drain itself through the earth connection. Ask for cleansing and know it is so. Dip your hands in salt water. Repeat the protection mantra: Let nothing but good come to me, nothing but good go from me. At home that night, you may want to bathe in soothing bath salts or mixture of Epsom salts and a drop of lavender and peppermint.

Your Reiki attunements will protect you, but, I believe, more deliberate protection engages you with the protection process and keeps you responsible for your own actions.

Because, as energy workers we are more susceptible, we can take on and ingest negative energy from food and drink. Bless your food and all who have come in contact with it, in particular, food eaten in restaurants. Who knows if an angry cook has sautéed the veggies!

I had dinner in a home once where the cook was disturbed at the behavior of her daughters-in-law. Still, she insisted on cooking and refused any help. Just after dinner four of the twelve or so present took sick with headaches. I left in terrible pain. Two men took to their chairs and one woman went to bed! Ever read *Like Water for Chocolate* by Laura Esquirel? Energy transference through food is one of the themes of the story.

If the client is of a high vibration, then the energy vibrations that move through the healer must be high enough to meet the demand and the healers' systems will attempt to clear itself to that level to meet this need. With the client "calling for" energy, the healer's field is taxed, and the energy rebound will escalate as a direct result of the increased energy demand, causing clearing.

When our systems have experienced this higher level, they will struggle to remain at the higher level because they are resonating to a purer vibration of Life Force Energy. Our spiritual selves sense "home" and desire this connection. The body attempts to stay there and going back to the lower levels may create complaints from the physical body in the form of discomfort, headaches, stomach aches, flu-like symptoms, feeling out of touch or disconnected. So, stick with the illness and clear the level(s) that are surfacing.

As the healer facilitates more opportunities for the purer energy to move through, the energy fields become healthier, more fine-tuned and the healer becomes more susceptible to bombardments from outside influences. As we healers heal ourselves, we are becoming higher vibrational beings and thus are forced to manicure our personal energy grids on a more regular basis.

As healers we have volunteered to raise our vibrations to better experience the Life Force Energy, the spiritual connection on this earth plane, but we must be able to fit into the higher vibratory package. Now we must honor the being we have become and keep our vehicle operating smoothly. We must keep our cup full to experience the expanding bounty of the healing energy that flows through us. We must commit to working at healing ourselves in order that others may come to the well we provide, to give them optimal opportunity to experience and heal so that they, in turn, may pass it on to others.

Ask for healing, complete, and total healing, healing on a cellular level. Let us be the best we can be, be every bit of who we can be in this lifetime.

The healing comes one person at a time.
And it begins with self.

~ 6 ~
Description of symbols

With Reiki II you become privy to three sacred symbols each representing a certain energy vibration for specific areas of healing. For centuries, the symbols were kept secret. Today they are published but remain a sacred trust. There is a fervor of discussion concerning the symbols' publication you may research if you wish.

Know that: the symbols should not be exhibited for public display; that their power is accessible only through an attuned Reiki master; they cannot harm anyone or come to harm. Treat them as sacred and give them a place of honor in your thoughts and use.

The first symbol is the Cho-Ku-Rei. It is like a light switch in that it increases the flow of energy. The second symbol is the Sei-He-Kei which is used for emotional healing, and clearing. The Hon-Sha-Ze-Sho-Nen symbol is used for sending distance healing.

Symbols are representations, images used to trigger certain accepted associations. A rose is the universal symbol of love; the cross for Christianity; two fingers raised in a V represents peace. The words on this page are simple figures in a structured, standardized form. It is thus with the Reiki symbols. We are a society of symbolic reasoning. Look to advertising for multitudinous examples.

When you are learning the symbols: practice. Practice drawing the symbols over and over until they are as familiar as your name. Draw them using different colors, markers and pencils. While you are practicing be attentive to the details. While any mistake you make in drawing the symbol during a healing session will be corrected by your Spirit Guides, it is still best to give each drawing your best effort. Singing or chanting the symbols will bring them into play as will visualizing them, however, it is still important to be particular and precise in learning how to draw, see, and send them. The sounds fit the Mickey Mouse tune! It is a great way to learn how to pronounce them and become familiar with them. And wasn't there healing sent every time the Mouseketeers sang their song?

The more you work with the symbols the more comfortable and confident you will become. Soon they should become second nature and you will find them popping into your vision and into your thoughts. They are wonderful companions! Symbols will resonate different with each practitioner because of the levels of vibration accessed.

When doing Reiki healings, draw the symbols as instructions come to your mind to do so. You need not continue to draw the symbols, although I have done so in a mantra like chant to access a meditative state. I almost always draw the symbols before starting a Reiki session to call the energy in. I draw symbols over the back of clients before sweeping them. Upon occasion I draw them with a universal intention attached. I often will draw the symbol over the client if a certain one has been called on for the healing session. For example, if the client is working with a recurring situation use the Hon-Sha-Ze-Sho-Nen. If the client has had a dramatic emotional release or healing, place the Sei-He-Kei in their auric field to protect them and help them stay free from the issue returning.

Colors can be used with the symbols although it is not mandatory and again should be a decision you make with your intuitive directives and your Spirit Guide's advice. If you "see" a symbol with a color, by all means, use it. If you are more comfortable to cover someone with a blue symbol or a violet symbol, then trust your intuition.

For a more accurate understanding of the combined energy, learn the significance of colors as you incorporate them into your intentions and prayers.

The symbols can be drawn in your mind, with your tongue on the roof of your mouth, or with your fingers (use your thumb and middle finger together for a powerful energetic focus). When you use your hand to draw the symbols, visualize them coming through your palm chakra.

You can draw the symbols on specific areas such as an elbow, a knee. It can be used in chakra clearing or for clearing a blockage in a decided location. I have also drawn huge symbols over the whole body of a person on the table laying it down with my hands. You will soon learn to feel the difference in vibrations they make, see how effective they are and how much easier they can make your job as a healer.

Intoning the symbols three times brings the power of three, which is the power of the trinity, of creation, or manifestation. Three is such a powerful number in our culture. There are three lights in the traffic symbol, three bears, three blind mice, Mother + father = child, three branches of government.

Meditate on the inherent qualities of each symbol. Feel which one resonates with you. Almost everyone feels an affinity with a specific symbol. Learn to understand their capabilities and how they work with your particular energetic "brand" of healing.

Be creative. Use these symbols often. Play with them. *They can do no harm.* The worst they can do is speed up healing on some level and while that is oftentimes uncomfortable, it isn't such a terrible thing.

~ 7 ~
The power symbol

Focus all the Power of the Universe Here

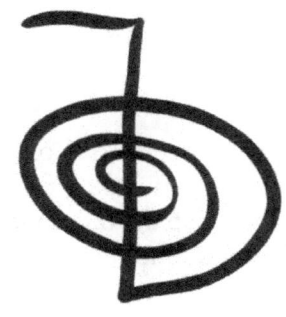

Cho-Ku-Rei

The **Cho-Ku-Rei** is the first symbol and is described as a light switch or power symbol. It increases the energy flow and thus the ability for healing to take place, in particular physical healing. William Rand explains that the top horizontal line represents universal ale energy, the down line symbolizes the energy coming to earth or the spinal column. The spiral, representing kundalini or female/earth energy crosses the spinal column 7 times - once for each of the primary chakras. The shape of this symbol is balanced. The left and right movement, the up and down movement, the spiraling circular movement all create balance. Line and circle cover all possibility of movement and the shape of the symbol covers all directional possibilities. What a wonder in such a tiny shape!

Drawing this symbol in a clockwise movement over a person, place or thing forces the energy inward, focusing and intensifying. Reversing the symbol or drawing it outward will help remove energy, pulling it out. Any block or negative energy will attach itself to the end of the spiral. It may come out like a ribbon or string.

I find the actual formation of the symbol to be very satisfying and peaceful. It is the one I resonate to. I find the spiral comforting and meditative. I look for spirals in nature and consider the symbolism of those objects. I try and relate these patterns back to the symbol and into my own life, at the moment of discovery. The connections you draw may prove fascinating.

I was once advised to do Cho-Ku-Reis over my belly chakra to increase my creative listening abilities. I was at a writer's retreat and was in the middle of a major revision of a novel. The Reiki Master working on me said to focus on the procreative, reproductive organs which are the source of biological creativity. At that same Reiki share I heard advice given to someone who was stuck on her path. She was told to visualize the symbol ahead of her footsteps as she walked and let the symbol support her movement forward.

Use this symbol to bring the energy in. If you are working on a specific pain, use this symbol to bring in more energy. If negative energy is difficult to remove, use this symbol to break up the blockage. Remember, everything is energy and energy vibrates at different rates, so anything you would like to see raised in vibration, cover with the power symbol. Reiki cannot harm. Increased vibrations will bring one and one's situations closer to pure, closer to enlightenment. More light and higher vibration may cause some lifestyle changes, but you will find those changes will be for the betterment of all concerned.

I have been cautioned about drawing this power symbol over a cancer. I suggest that you be very careful when drawing this symbol over a cancer, as cancer is exacerbated cellular growth. I also can reason that holding Reiki over the tumor will force its demise because it is not balanced with the flow of the body's true physical energy field. While I am convinced, beyond the shadow of doubt, that Reiki cannot harm, use your best judgment in this circumstance. You may want to switch to the emotional symbol and heal the emotions surrounding this disease.

38

I have been working with another energy therapist on a young man with cancer and the Reiki energy seems to be releasing some of the blockages surrounding the disease. And while I do not think the cancer will be cured, I believe the Reiki is bringing peace and easing the pain surrounding the disease. I caution you to be very conscious and aware of the strength of Reiki healing in all circumstances.

Use the Cho-Ku-Rei to clear a room. Draw it in the corners and on the ceiling and the floor. See the room as a box surrounded by increased light vibration.

Use this symbol on specific chakras to empower yourself in whatever area you may be struggling. For example, if you are going on a job interview or if you are approaching a discussion that is very important to you, Reiki your throat chakra so that your voice will ring true.

If you are struggling in a relationship on any level and need spiritual guidance, write the names of the people, places, and/or things on a piece of paper and draw the symbol on top. This will bring light and understanding and increased capabilities for your own discernment.

Using this symbol over your food in the form of a blessing will increase the nutritional effects and will negate any negatives surrounding the growth and preparation of the food.

Energize and purify the water you are drinking with this symbol. There are other methods of healing water on the Internet.

Use this symbol anywhere you want an increase in energy. When I pay my bills, I draw this symbol over my checks knowing that the energetic exchange does not exclude money.

Use it to speed up your computer.

Surround yourself with it when involved in a conversation where you wish to share wisdom and enlightenment with someone. (Remember that your truth may not be another's. Sharing is one thing, forcing your opinion on another is not loving or compassionate. Ask for words and wisdom.)

This symbol is easy to draw. It is easy to visualize. It is fun. It is easy to say. This tells me that Spirit wants this symbol used. With higher vibration, with more light coming to this planet (and it comes one person at a time) we will come faster to the true reality of our authentic selves and what our mission is here, and ultimately, I believe, to a more peaceful, loving way of life.

~ 8 ~
Mental-Emotional Symbol

God and Humanity become one.

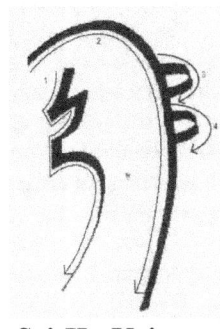

Sei-He-Kei

The Sei-He-Kei is used for emotional healing, for purification, protection, and clearing. It is used for releasing any emotional process if you suspect that physical distress is a direct result of an emotional concern. Physical manifestations cannot heal without healing the emotional factor, so focus on releasing old patterns of anger or limitations. Anger, jealousy, hate, depression, and fear are negative emotions that will not "hold" with the new vibration of Reiki II that you are now open to.

It is useful in relationships as relationships are our best teachers. A relationship is the result of two parties joining and so embodies the creative and manifesting power of three. It is here we learn about ourselves and how we relate to the world by the behavioral mirrors other people provide for us.

As taught by Don Miquel's Four Agreements, relationships are excellent vessels for learning to live without judgment, without taking on another's thoughts, words, or deeds. In any relationship the only person we can heal is ourselves and because we know every thought, word, and deed about ourselves, we become, often, the most difficult to forgive. Forgiving oneself is often the biggest single step in healing from emotional wounds. We expect so much from ourselves and do ourselves great damage by negative nagging. Forgive the fabulous, unique, beautiful person that is you.

Remember that relationships can be negative and sometimes the best way to heal them is to break the relationship. Some people are just not healthy for each other. Healing does not often look like our limited conclusions, so Let Go and Let Spirit be your guide. It is trust. It is faith.

The Sei-He-Kei reminds me of the end of a guitar and thus of music. Music is comfort and beauty and creativity. Music is relaxation, meditation, and dance.

This symbol can also be seen as a face. The left-hand side a nose and chin. The right side representing the cloak of Spirit guarding, covering and/or protecting.

William Rand sees the symbol as brain balance. The left side represents left brain and linear thinking with its angles and straight lines. He sees the curved right brain side as intuitive and imaginative thought.

Use two of these back-to-back when you are interested in creating harmony and balance although the use of a single symbol is a remarkable tool.

This symbol is fun and easy to draw. But be aware that emotional clearing is not always easy. Some tragic and traumatic events have occurred in people's lives. Reviewing and revisiting these events, even from an observer's standpoint, is not often pleasant. Necessary, I believe, but often not pleasant. I remind you again of lesson #289 from the Course in Miracles, "The past is over, it can touch me not." AND, you have Reiki to help heal any wound no matter how deep. In healing these wounds, I suggest you send healing to yourself, any other person and to the situation. Write the situation on a piece of paper and draw the symbol over it. This enhances the energy draw and with more energy to work with, the quicker healing can take place.

Use Reiki to assist your memory. For a test, draw the symbol over the test paper and pen. If you have lost something, draw the symbol over your head and ask for angelic help. I do this for a name or thought I have lost! Memory. You can also use this symbol with affirmations beginning with "I am" to further the strength of the symbol. I am taking the test with ease and have a high grade. I am reunited with my cell phone in one minute.

Use this symbol to cleanse a room of negative energy. Do the floor and ceiling and all four sides. I also suggest doing the doorways of any new places you enter so the negative can be dissipated.

I repeat this symbol often in healing when the emotional release has been substantial. Put it over the heart chakra, front and back. Draw it over any place damage has been done.

~ 9 ~
Distance symbol

The Spirit in me touches the Spirit in you.

The **Hon-Sha-Ze-Sho-Nen** is the symbol used for sending distance healing. Distance can be across miles and across time also. It is the symbol of past, present, future. Because of this it can aid in healing karmic behaviors, trends, and/or debts. This symbol must be drawn to send distance Reiki.

It is the most complicated of the five symbols and drawing it often causes the novice as well as the experienced practitioner much difficulty. That's okay. The difficulty is for a reason and the possibilities are numerous: To engage both sides of the brain so as not to take the symbol's power too lightly? To offer the user a challenge? To create thought and the opportunity to work through complexity? It is complicated to slow you down.

The symbol looks like a Pagoda, a tall stick house. The first part of the symbol draws nicely and flows but you will come to a part that creates a stumbling block. It causes you to stop and change direction. This hesitation, this change, perhaps eliminates lethargic recapitulations of this powerful symbol. It forces an abrupt shift mid-stream. It causes the user to forget where they are in the steps and forces a regrouping. All this creates an opportunity for practice and memorization which builds a user confidence and thus a confidence in these new

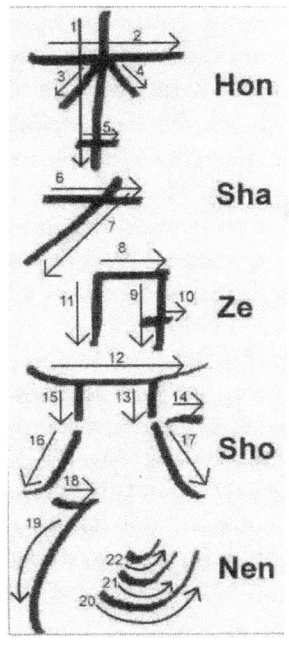

Hon

Sha

Ze

Sho

Nen

Hon-Sha.-Ze-Sho-Nen

healing abilities.

It also builds a relationship with this symbol that is frustrating, loving, challenging, and stimulating. Remember the ever presence of symbol-repair Spirit Guides! Keep practicing and keep using this remarkable symbol. I like to draw or say it three times to initiate the healing process.

This symbol is used to bless things and/or events that occur outside the present moment. Any event that causes you concern can receive a blessing. If the event is in the past, then healing energy, I believe, will ripple forward affecting every event that precedes it. In Star Trek the crew of the Enterprise had to be careful not to change the course of history with people and planets they came into contact with. But personally, we can change the events of our own lives in the past, present and future. Co-create your universe. Heal those things that have hurt you in this lifetime and in others. As you do, you work to heal your present moment and that, after all, is all we have!

Sending Reiki to future events gives a sense of Spiritual intervention leaving the sender more comfortable in the circumstance that has been blessed with Reiki energy. Send Reiki to the job interview, to the speech, the test, meeting your future mother-in-law, the hotel room in which you are booked, or to an airplane and the airport.

The distance symbol is used to work with people in transition. Those dying to this life experience will transition more easily with this symbol that bridges and covers all aspects of life.

Use also for spirits who are bound to the earth for some reason. Ghosts of entities who are trapped here. Remember, however, this is work that requires some knowledge and understanding way beyond this text, and these kinds of circumstances should be entered into with a knowledgeable person. Use this symbol to send them into the light. Work in love here. Only in love. Call on any Ascended Reiki Masters to come and assist you.

Send distance to those in your Reiki lineage. Send distance Reiki to the Ascended Masters. I do not know these souls by name, but I believe they are those who, while on the earth plane, worked with and mastered Reiki. We do know the names of some, Dr. Usui, Dr. Hayashi, Mrs. Takata. Perhaps you will become acquainted with some of these souls as Spirit Guides or Healing Guides.

These kinds of exercises in healing create a wonderful bond and understanding within the Reiki "family tree."

~10 ~
A Reiki treatment

A Sample Information Sheet for Clients

1) Reiki balances energies within and around the body. Its method of balancing the body's energies can be beneficial to people dealing with chronic pain, chronic illness, high stress, depression, anxiety, and emotional turmoil. Reiki operates on four levels of existence:

a) Physical – aids in balancing the energies of the body, assisting the body to heal itself in the process
b) Emotional – aids in balancing the emotional energies, assisting in understanding what the feelings are and how to come to terms with them
c) Mental – aids in balancing mental processes by opening possibilities to mind and body connections/relationships
d) Spiritual – aids in balancing spiritual energies, assisting in developing the capacity to love self and others

2) Reiki focuses on the cause rather than the effect of dis-ease. Instead of treating the symptoms independent of the cause, it affects the root cause of the disease. Reiki accelerates the natural healing process. Disease as we speak it and write it as one word can be sentencing and thus can become baggage. Written with a hyphen the word is broken down into its parts. Dis means the absence of; ease refers to "the condition of being comfortable or relieved, freedom from pain, worry or agitation (The American Heritage College Dictionary pg 394, 431). Dis-ease then is merely the absence of comfort and so becomes much easier to work with in terms of energy release.

3) **Clients** often report the following reaction during a Reiki treatment:
   a. Seeing colors or feeling serenity while the energy flows through the body
   b. Feeling very relaxed as the energy flows
   c. Some people will fall asleep
   d. Feeling peace and/or strong emotions as old patterns or memories surface
   e. Feeling a shift of consciousness. This is an important part of the healing process.

4) **What should** the client do to prepare for a treatment?
   a. Take off shoes, watch, and cumbersome jewelry.
   b. Relax and enjoy the balance.

5) **What does** the Reiki practitioner do during a treatment?
   a. A Reiki practitioner works with the energy centers and any areas of specific pain in the body.
   b. A practitioner will make the space as comfortable and as relaxing as possible. Music. Pillows.
   c. A practitioner will help release thoughts and fears so the client can focus on the moment, the present, and the experience. This is done by breathing or by speaking if the client is comfortable sharing their concerns.

6) **After the treatment:**
   a. Some people will feel energized.
   b. Most feel an incredible sense of relaxation and peace.

DRINK WATER. It is recommended to drink six 8-ounce glasses of water each day for three days after the balance. Water flushes toxins that are loosened during treatment. Water is very important to the overall health of the body, mind and spirit.

Getting in touch with the subtle energies of the body may cause you to examine some of the habits and lifestyle choices you make in determining more healthful, positive modifications.

Some practitioners will recommend scheduling another appointment to continue the healing process and to maintain wellness. Long standing difficulties often take multiple treatments to access and treat deep-seated causes. In general, the more long-standing the difficulty, the more Reiki energy will be needed to achieve the highest benefit. Holding onto physical distress becomes a way of life for some and while pain may be uncomfortable, we learn how to adapt to it and live with it. For this reason, complete and immediate removal of the pain is often too much for a client to adjust to quickly. The best way to remove deep-seated distress is to remove it a layer at a time. The mental and emotional bodies then have a chance to adjust and shift with the changes in the physical body.

~ 11 ~
An energy balance

There is no separation. Not from each other, not from God,
and not from anything that is…
Act as if you were separate from nothing, and no one,
and you will heal your world tomorrow.

Walsch, *Conversations with God,* Book 3, 44

Because many of you reading this will be working with others who include other energy healing modalities with their Reiki balance, I include this method of balance for your information and consideration. This may seem complicated, but it is nothing you are asked to memorize and adhere to for each balance you preform. It is how I work because I like to be involved with the energy. I like to participate.

I believe that you can sit with your hands on any part of a person's body and the Reiki will flow to where it is needed. You can also place your hands above each chakra, front and back, and the healing will take place.

I believe the best thing to do sometimes is to take yourself as far out of the healing as possible. Go to the zone and meditate while the energy runs through you. This eliminates the control issue and any judgments that may surface. It is also a wonderful way to enjoy the healing that runs through you to your client.

Practice your Reiki balances the way they are most comfortable for you. Use these suggestions as required for each balance.

Do not be concerned that you will be faced with a situation that is more than you can handle. Spirit knows and will not overburden or place you in a situation that you are not prepared for. We are not all counselors, but we are volunteers in the healing energy team! Spirit is not looking for us to fail a client, but to "use" us to facilitate the healing.

There is no ritual to follow. Every balance is different. The following are suggestions as to methods and processes you may accept or reject as you are guided.

State your invocation prayer asking the energy to flow and inviting your Guides to work beside and through you. I suggest you say the Reiki symbols three times. The symbols will flow into use, but working intentionally with them will increase your understanding of their abilities.

The client may want a pillow under their feet or head. Be sure they are warm enough. They should lay with their feet uncrossed and arms at their sides.

Taking a few deep, belly breathes together will help center each of you and create a connection. I like to do a count of eight inhaling, holding, and exhaling.

With hands 3-4 inches above the body, in the physical/emotional section of the aura, do a general scan to get the Chi lines running. Notice any hot spots that will need direct attention. Scan the kundalini line (the spine or center meridian) and the sides of the body.

Check for hot spots in higher layers of the aura by lifting your hands up and through the layers. Layers collapsing one onto the other can cause a person to feel sluggish, heavy, or lethargic. This upward sweeping movement of your hands through the various fields will act as a comb through the auric field. The healing, positive energy in your hands will attract any negative energy blockages causing them to dissipate the same way as when the hands are placed on the physical body. Auras are expansive and need to be such. Pulling your hands up and through the aura if you feel the need will open lines up through the aura and separate any layers lying to close together.

Collapsing auric layers will often feel like sludge and the upward movement may be hindered because the energy is thick. Fluffing the aura, spinning your hands around in a combing movement will often help this as well, as deep breaths from the client force a rod of light through the center of their trunk.

Check each chakra to insure it is open and sustaining an unhindered flow of energy. The chakras will spin. The direction of the spin does not matter, the body will adjust that. You can lift the energy, like a vortex, up from the chakra, up through the aura. In a gentle motion, twist your flat hand up and out in a spiraling manner, widening and increasing the rotations as you spin and lift. Often energy blocks will attach themselves to you while you are working out in the auric field. You can follow them down to the block. Pick them up and pull them up and out through the layers. This may take several attempts. Hold your hands over the position to put "clean" energy back into the now free place. This may take 5-10 minutes over each chakra. The flow of the energy will ebb when it is time to move on.

For additional chakra work you can visualize the chakra system as a line in the center of the body. Put your hands flat over the center of the body, pointer fingers and thumbs together to create a triangle. Or with hands vertical, flat over the body point the energy finger (the pointer) down at a right angle. Either position, moving up and down the center line, will help align the chakras. The hand's energy becomes a vacuum cleaner attachment pulling from all the energy centers at once and balances each.

Be sure to check the palm chakras, in particular with people who say they always have cold hands. Cold hands = blockage. Work on the shoulders may help to open the hands. You can create an energy line by putting your energy finger (tall man/middle finger) in the center of the palm chakra of the client and atop the shoulder at the point where the bones meet. Hold until you feel the energy between your hands. Then you can collapse this line by moving your hands closer together by moving the hand on the shoulder down the center of the arm to the inside center of the elbow. Collapse further to the wrist and the palm.

If the palm chakra is difficult to open, massage between the wrists and the forearms. Massage the hands between the bones. In a gentle but firm motion, pull the fingers outward. Be sure to hold the client's hand steady so that they do not have to be conscious of holding for you to work on. They should be by this time relaxed and trusting of the energy and the workers, so do not force them out of this state.

Before you turn the client over have them do some breathing, breathing up and down from crown to foot and vice versa to ground and remove energy residue. The client's breath should be greater now, expanding the muscles of the chest cavity and lifting the stomach off the table, then forcing the stomach back to the spine on the out breath.

Comb the auric field again and draw any symbols as you are led to do so. Sweep this side of the client to remove residue. Sweeping the client is a simple brushing movement from head to toe and pushing outward or downward to brush and cleanse this side. Save the Raku movement for when you are finished.

Speak to the client, without startling them. They may be asleep! Remember they are in a very vulnerable state here with the front balanced and not the back. Ask them to turn over. Be sure they are comfortable when they get settled in, face down on the table. They may need pillows under their feet for support. Be sure their feet are not crossed and try to get them to lie with their hands upright (arms flat on the table) so you can recheck the palm chakras and the energy running down the arm.

Work on the back is often the time clients are most relaxed. They often sleep or are in a "zone" state of peace and harmony. Honor their space and the quiet of the moment. This is a good time for you to "zone" also.

Run energy from crown to feet. Have the client do a few deep breaths. Work up and down the body in the same way as you did the front and wherever else you are directed.

Work now on the back of the head and neck. You can press the pressure points at the base of the cranium – often called the Voice of God – and work the soft tissue around the neck vertebrae. You can check an acupressure point chart for exact location. I also like to work the ears here, putting our palm over the client's ears.

A good position is to place a hand at each end of the spine and run energy up and down. You may feel led to put your hand at the top of the crown and the base of the spine. Watch touching the client where they may be uncomfortable.

Pay particular attention to the shoulder blades. These are important pressure points. It seems to be a good "storage" spot for stress and often the energy block will radiate to the neck and/or back and can cause headaches. Women tend to "shoulder" many responsibilities and often have energy blocked here.

Check all the chakra points as they have openings in the back also. Do not forget to check the minor chakras in the joints. Check the backs of the knees.

Working on the legs and feet, collapse the energy line from hip to foot, back of the knee to foot, to work the energy down the leg line.

In coming to the close of the balance, comb the auric field again to check for free movement. Draw symbols in the aura as you are guided before finishing. If the healing has facilitated a lot of emotional release, then I suggest the Sei-He-Kei to protect. If the healing has been for a client very low in energy, the Cho-Ku-Rei in their aura will give them an energetic boost long past the time they get off the table. One book I read says to put the Sei-He-Kei in the solar plexus for lengthening the healing effects. Go with your intuition here and trust your heart and thought. Ask your Guides for advice on what is best.

Hold the client for a moment in sacred space. Go into deep prayer with their best intentions as a focus. Thank all the Guides who have been present for the healing. This time of extending gratitude is an excellent way to bring closure to the healing time. Remember, the client honors and trusts you by inviting you into their aura and their spiritual space.

Separate yourself from the client by drawing the Raku in front of your heart.

Sweep the auric field of the client either with a smooth hand movement from the crown to the feet or zig-zagging the Raku down the client to block and separate.

Sweeping is to come from the head to the feet of the client in a Raku, a zig-zag movement, much alike a lightning bolt. I use the Raku for separation between the client and the release and between the client and the healer.

Advise the client to get up slowly. Sit with them a minute to see if they are okay. I like to excuse myself to go and wash my hands while they get their thoughts together and their shoes on.

Remind them to **DRINK WATER**, lots of water, as toxins will need to flush. The healing will continue for the next three days. Water will facilitate an easier flow of release and replenish the body.

WASH YOUR HANDS or clean them in the heat of a candle.

Answer questions. Set another appointment if you feel it is advisable. I prefer to do three visits close together when I begin working with a new client, once a week or every other week. This gives the body time to adjust to the stages of release and free-flowing energy. This also helps the client grasp a better feeling and understanding of the process.

The energy you are channeling to the client will work itself to every place it needs to be for the moment. If you sit at the crown chakra and channel healing for an hour the client's body will get appropriate healing!

While the movements and procedures are designed to facilitate easy and quick healing and to assist the body, any hands-down position will work. Stressing yourself over proper healing techniques hinders the flow of pure Spirit because your own fears will use the energy. Visualize yourself as a pipeline. If your pipe is corroded with old belief patterns and fears, then where is the healing going to take place? On the first place it finds a need. So, clearing yourself of hindrances on all levels assists others you work on/with.

~ 12 ~
New Reiki information

Reissuing the *In Touch With Reiki I, II, and III Manuals for Students/Teachers* gives me cause to reflect on the ever growing importance of Reiki in my life, giving me an amazing sense of self-strength and capability to travel through the experiences of my life. Reiki is my lifeline, my anchor, my launch pad!

What I know is that Reiki supports any additional healing modality, enhances all innate talents, and gives support when looking at issues as an involved participant or as an observer. What I will share is how I learned to let go and allow the Reiki energy to flow and heal with its own wisdom.

One of my greatest lessons has been with my friend I will call Tomi. Tomi and I worked in a small doctor's office together as receptionists. She was diagnosed with breast cancer during her second pregnancy, age 27. It took this conservative Baptist woman a bit to say yes to my invitations to try Reiki yet when she did, she loved the relaxation it brought her.

We did not have much time for Reiki as Tomi was a mother and wife, working full-time while struggling with chemo and radiation. We set up a twin bed in a spare room in the office where we'd "work" in 15–25-minute stints on lunch hours and occasionally before 8am. With so limited time and space, I did not work the chakras or concern myself with any hand positions. I sat at the head of the bed with a pillow and Tomi's head on my lap. I worked with Archangel Gabriel because

Tomi named the child she was carrying at the time of her diagnosis Gabriel.

As Tomi learned to relax into the energy, we would "disappear" into the healing process. I learned to completely trust the linear time passage because at the perfect time, every time, we would both come "back." The Reiki took her to a safe, pain free state of no fear. Until... Tomi began to feel the Reiki was causing her more pain when the session was over than the tranquil state was beneficial. I believe she began to leave her body during these sessions. I could not get her to understand that concept. I was conflicted, struggling to understand why the Reiki was hurting her and that I could no longer use it to help her through her illness and make the cancer go away. So I stopped putting my hands directly on her and I began to send distance Reiki to her surroundings. And her condition continued to worsen.

As I struggled with all this, a colleague told me that by putting my hands on Tomi's head where the cancer had metastasized, I was feeding the cancer. I completely freaked out until after much research, prayer, and many consultations with other energetic healers and Reiki practitioners, I became, and continue to be, 100% convinced that Reiki cannot do harm. My intentions for her healing were pure. They were colored by my egoistic desire, a human limitation embossed with much love for my friend. I believe the energy does what it is guided to do by the person receiving the energy and that neither my ego nor my belief system could interfere with that. And, I believe I am forgiven, excused and blessed, as I continue to learn and grow in understanding the nature of Reiki energy and of living without trying to control and/ or judge.

My lesson in this was twofold. First, it was my adamant desire, hope, prayer, wish, and intention that Tomi regain perfect health. I believe this is what she wanted, and I believe she took her life contract to the foot of God to plead her case. She wanted to stay and raise her children, do her job, live this lifetime. It was not to be. And, I had to completely let go of the outcome and allow Tomi her relationship with her experience; not judge God; keep my own faith, not only in God, but faith in my own energetic capabilities and limitations.

As a result of that experience, I have decreased the number of hand positions I use during most of my healing sessions. Because people allow themselves so little down time and put themselves under so much pressure, I like for them to be as quiet and still for as long as possible. So, I have them lay face up on the table the whole session, no longer having them turn over to work on their back chakras.

First, I place my hands under the person's head for, sometimes, 30 minutes of the whole session. I cup their skull with my fingers at the base of their skull. So often headaches are felt here, and stress so easily finds its way here. Fingers pressing on the base of the skull is, well, my two-year client says, is the very best and moans her discontent every time I take my hands away, no matter how long I have stayed on this position! She says she feels the energy working through her whole body from this position and is able to connect with it.

Then I move to their side and place one hand under the person's neck and the other under the base of their spine. I call this the cradle position. To lie in it feels like you are wrapped in warmth, love and safety. I believe this position works in all of the chakras. If I find one or another chakra needs attention, I can blow the symbols of healing into it. Or I can use my eyes to send healing, or I ask my guides to handle that spot.

Next, I will hold the adrenals to release toxins by placing one hand just under their hip and the other on their side almost like my hands are in a 90-degree angle. Many people do not like their belly touched but touching their side seems to be okay. I will often switch hands at the same position to refill any energetic release with healing Reiki.

Then I hold the relaxed person's feet to ground them back in. If they have gone deep into the session, I will brush their legs, physically touching them, from the knees to the feet, three or four times. Then I do the usual aura sweeping. I tap them on the shoulder to let them know the session is complete. I leave the room to cleanse my hands so they can fully "return." I bring them a glass of water to remind them that drinking plenty of water further facilitates the healing over the next few days.

At one point in my Reiki career (for many years) I wanted to know, see, and/or hear the energies at work. I wanted to understand what the person was releasing, how it was affecting their body. After all, lots of my companions could see it, feel it, hear it and I wanted to, too! But, I don't. Yet, I have grown to be very content in accepting my personal gifts. I believe I am most competent when I completely step out of the way of the process, disappear into the moment, and let the energies do their calling. It is simply my responsibility to be the most clear and unbiased Reiki channel I can be.

The Reiki process is between the energy and the receiver! And I am finally content and confident in allowing that to happen and simply being a part of the moment.

I encourage you to respect and honor the unique and individual Reiki practitioner that you are and that you will grow into. Be your blessed self and accept your uniqueness.

~ 13 ~
The Reiki Principles

Just for today, do not anger.
Just for today, do not worry.
We shall count our blessings and honor our fathers
and mothers, our teachers and neighbors and honor our food.
Make an honest living.
Be kind to everything that has life.

Hawayo Takata,
The History of Reiki as Told by Mrs. Takata

Just for today do not worry.
Just for today do not anger.
Honor your parents, teachers and elders.
Earn your living honestly.
Show gratitude to everything.
Respect the Oneness of All Life.

Diane Stein, *Essential Reiki*

Just for today, I will live in the attitude of gratitude.
Just for today, I will not worry.
Just for today, I will not anger.
Just for today, I will do my work honestly.
Just for today, I will show love and respect for every human being.

Paula Horan, *Empowerment through Reiki*

These are words we can aspire to. They remind us to live in the now, to love all of life. It is so simple and yet it is so difficult at times. Live from moment to moment and if you fall off the love-everything wagon, work towards forgiving yourself and all others involved and move on. Just for today. Just for the moment, because this moment is all we have!

~ Bibliography ~

Course in Miracles. Foundation for Inner Peace, 1992.

The American Heritage College Dictionary. 3rd Edition. Boston: Houghton, Mifflin Co, 1993.

Andrew, Elizabeth. *Writing the Sacred Journey: The Art and Practice of Spiritual Memoir.* Skinner House Books. Boston, MA, 2005.

Angelo, Jack. *Hands on Healing.* Rochester, VT: Healing Arts Press, 1994.

Baginski, Bodo J and Shalila Sharamon. *Reiki Universal Life Energy.* Mendocino, CA Life Rhythm, 1988.

Bourbeau, Lise. *Listen to Your Body.* Saint-Sauveur des Monts (Quebec), Editions E.T.C. Inc, 1989.

Bourbeau, Lise. *Heal Your Wounds and Find Your True Self.* Saint-Sauveur des Monts (Quebec), Editions E.T.C. Inc, 2001.

Bourbeau, Lise. *Your Body's Telling You: Love Yourself!* Saint-Sauveur des Monts (Quebec), Editions E.T.C. Inc, 2001.

Bradford, Michael. *The Healing Energy of Your Hands.* Freedom, CA, The Crossings Press, 1993.

Burnham, Sophy. *The Ecstatic Journey.* New York, NY: Ballantine Books, 1977.

Carter, Karen Rauch. *Move Your Stuff, Change Your Life.* New York, NY: Fireside, 2000.

Emerson, Barbara. *Self-Healing Reiki.* Berkeley, CA: Frog, LTD, 2001.

Esquivel, Laura. *Like Water for Chocolate.* New York, NY: Random House. 1992

Fuentes, Star. *Light Language - Beginner's Manual.* 1992.

Garfield, Charles, Cindy Spring and Sedonia Cahill, *Wisdom Circles.* New York, NY, Hyperion, 1998.

Hay, Louise L., *Heal Your Body.* Carson, CA, The Hay House, 1982.

Herman, Deborah Levine with Cynthia Black. *Spiritual Writing.* Hillsboro, OR, Beyond Words Publishing, Inc., 2002.

Horan, Paula, *Empowerment through Reiki.* Twin Lakes, WI, Lotus Light-Shangri-La, 1996.

Horan, Paula. *Abundance through Reiki.* Twin Lakes, WI, Lotus Light-Shangri-La, 1995.

International Association of Reiki Professionals, www.iarp.org.

The "I AM" Discourses. St Germain Foundation Schamburg, IL, St Germain Press, 1996.

Mitchell, Karyn. Reiki: *A Torch in Daylight.* St. Charles, IL, Mind River Publications, 1994.

Motz, Julie. *Hands of Life.* New York, NY: Bantam Books. 1998.

Narrin, Janeanne. *One Degree Beyond.* Seattle, WA, Little White Buffalo Publishing Cottage, 1998.

NumberQuest - http://numberquest.com/numbers.html

Petter, Frank Arjava. *Reiki Fire.* Twin Lakes, WI, Lotus Light- Shangri-La, 1997.

Petter, Frank Arjava. *The Original Reiki Handbook of Dr. Mikao Usui.* Twin Lakes, WI: Lotus Light Shangri-La, 1999.

Ponder, Catherine. *Open Your Mind to Prosperity.* Marina del Rey, CA, DeVorss and Co., 1971.

Ponder, Catherine. *The Dynamic Laws of Healing.* Marina del Rey, CA, DeVorss and Company, 1966.

Rand, William. Reiki - *The Healing Touch.* First and Second Degree Manual. Southfield, MI, Vision Publications. 1998.

Redfield, James. *Celestine Prophecy.* New York, NY, Warner Books, Inc., 1997.

Ruiz, Don Miguel. *The Four Agreements.* San Rafael, CA, AmberAllenPublishing,1997. http://www.miguelruiz.com/agreements.html

Sai Baba Workshop booklet.

Shin, Florence Shovel. *The Game of Life and How to Play It.* Marina del Rey, CA, DeVorss, 1925.

Stein, Diane. *Essential Reiki.* 4th printing. Freedom, CA, The Crossings Press, 1996.

Suess, Dr., *Green Eggs and Ham.* New York, NY, Random House, 1988.

Thayer, Steven and Linda Sue Nathanson, *Interview with an Angel.* Gillette, NJ, Edin Books, 1997.

Twyman, James. E-site James@emissaryoflight.com

Unity Publications. *Daily Word.* Unity Worldwide Ministries, Unity Village, MO,

Walsch, Neale Donald, *Conversations with God.* Book 1. Charlottesville, VA, Hampton Roads, 1996.

Walsch, Neale Donald, *Conversations with God.* Book 2. Charlottesville, VA, Hampton Roads, 1997.

Walsch, Neale Donald, *Conversations with God.* Book 3. Charlottesville, VA, Hampton Roads, 1998.

Walsch, Neale Donald, *Friendship with God.* New York, NY, G. P. Putman's Sons, 1999.

Williamson, Marianne. *A Return to Love.* New York, NY, HarperPerennial, 1992.

Zukav, Gary. *Seat of the Soul.* New York, NY, Fireside, Simon and Schuster, 1998.

There are many wonderful Reiki books available. And many more on healing and self-development. I encourage you to seek Spiritual connection through the written word. Reading helps you to connect with other's experiences and thoughts. Remain free to accept or reject any thought that does not resonate with the truth you feel in your soul. Rejecting often solidifies your own beliefs. Explaining yourself helps solidify your truths and so you are free to grow and explore and expand.

About the Author

Susan Rea Caldwell, MA, RM, wears many hats. She received her BA from the University of Kentucky in 1994 and in 1996 her MA from Marshall University in English and Creative Writing.

As a writer she has received several grants from the Kentucky Foundation for Women, has published many short stories and two novels, *Betty Rea and Joseph's Journey*, a collection of vignettes, *Tales from smack in the middle of New Hampshire Drive and a few miles beyond: The Gordon and Ivan series.*

She has practiced energy balance therapy since 1996 when becoming a Usui Reiki Master/Teacher. She has written manuals for each level of Reiki training, *In Touch with Reiki - Manuals for Teachers and Students, Levels I, II, III.*

Susan is an Akashic Records consultant, guiding a client through a dialogue with the keepers of the events of their soul's personal journey.

As a labyrinth facilitator, certified through Veriditas@ she leads labyrinth walks for personal healing, for global healing, for guidance and direction, and for expanding creativity.

As a workshop leader she facilitates Julia Cameron's Artist's Way providing intense and gratifying path for seekers on their path to personal truth. She also hosts play shops in making prayer flags and vision boards.

As an artist, Susan creates fabric collage wall hangings using repurposed and vintage items, particularly hand-crafted items.